Guided Imagery for Healing

Guided Imagery for Healing

The science and practice of guided imagery for relaxation, surgery preparation, and healing.

Becky Stevens, MSN, CRNA, HWNC-BC, CA

Photo of the author by Leticia London

All other images courtesy of Canva.com

ISBN-13: 979-8-9930692-1-0

E-book ISBN-13: 979-8-9930692-0-3

Library of Congress Control Number: 2025919284

Becky Stevens & Co., LLC

Published in the United States of America

This book is dedicated to my patients, all of whom have been my best teachers.

Table of Contents

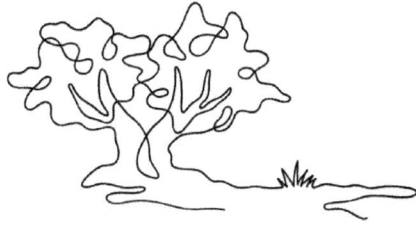

"The mind is everything. What you think you become."

-Buddha

Introduction

If you're preparing for surgery, recovering from illness or injury, or simply looking for ways to support your body's natural healing processes, you may already know that your mind plays a powerful role in your health and healing. You've already experienced it yourself — when you're stressed, your heart races, your muscles tense, and your sleep suffers. But when you feel safe and at ease, your breathing slows, your body relaxes, your mind is clear, and you have more energy.

Guided imagery is a simple yet powerful way to tap into your mind's ability to influence your body. It's a practice that uses your imagination — along with all of your senses — to create calming, healing experiences in your mind that have real effects on your physical and emotional well-being.

For decades, researchers, healthcare providers, and therapists have used guided imagery to help patients prepare for surgery, manage pain, recover more quickly, and reduce anxiety before and after medical procedures. The beauty of guided imagery is that it's safe, gentle, non-invasive, and something you can do anywhere — in a quiet room, in your hospital bed, or in a waiting area before a procedure or appointment.

This book is your companion for learning, practicing, and using guided imagery to support healing. You don't need to be "good at meditation," have any special skills, or believe in anything mystical. All that's required is an open mind and a willingness to practice.

How to Use This Book

In this book, you'll find:

- A clear explanation of what guided imagery is and how it works.

- Research-based information about the benefits and limitations of guided imagery.

- Step-by-step guidance for practicing imagery with audio or on your own.

- Scripts for specific situations, from general healing to preparing for surgery or getting through a quick medical procedure.

- Ideas for complementary practices like relaxation, music, aromatherapy, and affirmations.

- Resources and references for further exploration.

- Each part contains summaries for quick review and reflection questions, inviting you to pause and engage more deeply.

By the end, you'll have the tools you need to use guided imagery as part of your healing journey with comfort and confidence.

Part I – Understanding Guided Imagery

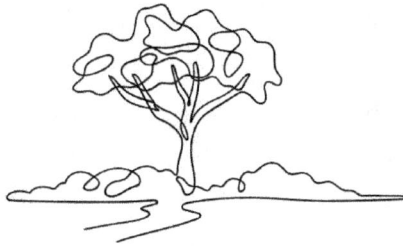

"Every thought we think is creating our future."

-Louise Hay

Chapter 1 – What Is Guided Imagery?

Imagine yourself lying in bed the night before your surgery: you close your eyes, take a slow, deep breath, and picture yourself walking along a quiet beach at sunrise. You see clouds floating and birds soaring in the sky, feel the warmth of the sun on your face, hear the gentle rhythm of the waves, and smell the salt in the air. Your body is strong and healthy, and you feel calm and at peace. When you awaken in the morning, you feel rested and relaxed. You know that you are well-prepared for your surgery, that you will have a positive experience, and that your body is ready to heal.

That's guided imagery in action — intentionally creating mental pictures and sensations that promote relaxation, well-being, and healing.

A Simple Definition

Guided imagery is a focused relaxation technique that uses all of your senses to create positive images and experiences in your mind. It's called "guided" because you typically follow a script, recording, or live facilitator who leads you through the process.

Guided imagery is similar to daydreaming — but with a purpose. You're not just letting your mind wander; you're directing it toward scenes, sensations, and experiences that help your body and mind work together for your benefit.

How It Compares to Other Practices

Meditation often focuses on clearing the mind or staying present with sensations; guided imagery invites you to create vivid mental experiences.

Hypnosis involves a different depth of trance and may use formal suggestions; guided imagery can be looser, lighter, and more conversational.

Visualization is closely related, but guided imagery emphasizes using all the senses — not just "seeing" in your mind.

Where It Comes From

Humans have used imagery for thousands of years in healing traditions, rituals, and spiritual practices. Modern guided imagery as a health tool emerged in the 1970s and 1980s, when mind-body medicine gained momentum. Today, it's used in hospitals, cancer centers, rehabilitation programs, and wellness settings around the world.

Why It's Used in Healing

Guided imagery helps by:

- Reducing anxiety before medical procedures

- Promoting relaxation and restful sleep

- Supporting pain management

- Encouraging positive expectations for recovery

- Helping you feel more in control during medical treatment

Even if your body is dealing with surgery or illness, your mind can create experiences of safety, comfort, and healing — and those experiences can influence how your body responds.

Chapter 2 – How Guided Imagery Works

Guided imagery might feel like "just using your imagination," but your body doesn't treat it that way. When you picture a scene vividly enough — imagining sights, sounds, smells, textures, and emotions — your brain responds as if you were really there. Those signals don't just stay in your head; they ripple throughout your body, affecting your heart rate, breathing, hormones, and even your immune system.

The Mind-Body Connection

The mind-body connection is the constant two-way communication between what we call the body - our physical state and functions, and what we call the mind - our thoughts, feelings, moods, and beliefs. Thoughts, images, and feelings send chemical and electrical signals through your nervous system and bloodstream. This connection is why your heart races when you're scared, or your jaw and shoulders tighten when you're stressed.

Guided imagery taps into this same system, but with intention. By creating calm, healing images, you send your body messages of safety and comfort — and these messages shift your nervous system into a more relaxed, balanced state.

The Relaxation Response

When you feel safe and at ease, your body activates the parasympathetic nervous system — also known as the "rest and digest" response. This is the opposite of the sympathetic nervous system, or the "fight or flight" response you experience during stress.

The relaxation response:

- Slows your heart rate

- Lowers blood pressure

- Eases muscle tension

- Improves digestion and circulation

- Balances stress hormones

Guided imagery can trigger this response in just a few minutes, even in the midst of a busy hospital or clinic setting. And the more you practice, the better and faster your body learns to shift into this healing mode.

Influencing the Brain

Modern brain imaging studies show that guided imagery activates the same brain regions you use when having an actual experience:

- The visual cortex lights up when you imagine seeing.

- The auditory cortex responds when you imagine sounds.

- The motor cortex activates when you imagine movement.

Practicing guided imagery is like a rehearsal for your brain and your body. For surgical patients, imagery of a smooth, successful procedure and rapid recovery can help create positive expectations — and where your mind goes, your body follows.

Supporting the Immune System

Research in psychoneuroimmunology — the study of how thoughts and emotions affect immunity — shows that reducing stress can help your immune system work more effectively. Some studies suggest that guided imagery may:

- Increase certain immune cell activity

- Improve wound healing

- Reduce markers of inflammation

While imagery isn't a magic cure, it can be a supportive partner to medical treatment, creating conditions in your body that make healing more likely.

Pain Modulation

Pain isn't just a physical signal; it's shaped by your brain's interpretation of those signals. Guided imagery can help you manage pain by:

- Redirecting your focus away from discomfort

- Replacing pain-related images with calming or neutral ones

- Reducing muscle tension that makes pain worse

- Helping you feel more in control, which can lower perception and improve tolerance of pain

The "Healing Blueprint" Concept

Some guided imagery experts describe it this way: when you create a clear mental picture of health and healing, you're giving your body a blueprint to work toward. Your nervous system, immune system, and endocrine system all receive the message that repair and recovery are the priority.

In the next chapter, we'll explore what the research shows about guided imagery — from reducing anxiety before surgery, to easing pain afterward, to supporting wound healing. You'll see where the evidence is strong, where it's still emerging, and what that means for you as you begin your own practice.

Chapter 3 – Benefits and Applications

You now know that guided imagery can create real changes in your body by calming your nervous system, shifting your focus, and influencing brain and immune function. But what does that look like in real life?

Over the years, guided imagery has been used in hospitals, rehabilitation centers, cancer clinics, sports medicine, and wellness programs — often with encouraging results. While guided imagery is not a substitute for medical care, it is a powerful complement to standard medical treatment that promotes self-care and active participation.

Let's look at some of the most common ways guided imagery can help.

Preparing for Surgery

Facing surgery often stirs up a mix of emotions: fear, anxiety, hope, and sometimes even excitement about getting relief from a problem. Guided imagery can help you feel more grounded and confident going in.

How it helps:

- Reduces preoperative anxiety

- Helps you mentally rehearse a smooth, safe procedure

- Encourages trust in your medical team and your body's ability to heal

- Can improve sleep quality (important both before surgery and during recovery)

- May reduce the need for medications, including sedatives, narcotics, and anti-hypertensives

Example:

Before her knee replacement, Maria listened to a 15-minute "successful surgery" imagery every night. She imagined the operating room as a place of safety, her surgeon working skillfully, and her body responding beautifully to the procedure. On the day of surgery, she reported feeling calm and ready. She woke up feeling well, and her anesthetist commented that her vital signs remained stable throughout the procedure.

Supporting Recovery After Surgery

Once the surgery is over, guided imagery can help you focus your energy on healing.

How it helps:

- Promotes relaxation, which supports tissue repair

- Can reduce the perception of pain

- May shorten recovery time and length of hospital stay

- Encourages gentle movement and confidence during rehabilitation

- Helps with sleep and energy restoration

Easing Pain

Pain is more than just a physical sensation — it's shaped by attention, emotion, and memory. Guided imagery can interrupt the cycle of tension and fear that can make pain worse.

How it helps:

- Shifts focus away from discomfort

- Uses calming mental images to soften the perception of pain

- Reduces muscle tension and stress hormones that intensify pain

- Gives you a sense of control, which can reduce distress

Managing Anxiety and Stress

Even when you're not facing surgery, guided imagery can be a gentle way to manage anxiety, whether it's related to illness, injury, or everyday life.

How it helps:

- Calms the "fight or flight" response

- Brings your awareness to the present moment

- Creates feelings of safety and ease

- May improve mood and outlook over time

Enhancing Recovery from Illness or Injury

Healing from illness or injury often takes patience. Guided imagery can help you stay positive and connected to your body's healing process.

How it helps:

- Encourages positive expectations

- Reinforces healthy behaviors like rest, hydration, and gentle activity

- Supports immune function during recovery

- Can help you feel more engaged and hopeful

Living Well with Chronic Conditions

For people managing chronic illness, guided imagery can be an ongoing tool for comfort, motivation, and resilience.

How it helps:

- Offers daily stress relief

- Improves coping skills

- Helps manage symptoms like fatigue or insomnia

- Supports emotional well-being

Complementary Use in Rehabilitation and Wellness

Guided imagery is often used alongside:

- Physical therapy (imagining muscles and joints working smoothly)

- Athletic training (visualizing performance and recovery)

- Wellness routines (combining with yoga, mindfulness, or breathing exercises)

A Gentle Reminder

While guided imagery can be a helpful partner in healing, it's not a replacement for medical treatment. Think of it as a tool in your self-care toolbox — one that works best when combined with your doctor's guidance, a healthy lifestyle, and the treatments you need.

In the next chapter, we'll take a closer look at what the research actually says about guided imagery — from the strongest evidence to where more studies are needed — so you can understand its benefits with a clear, informed perspective.

Part I Summary

In these opening chapters, we've explored what guided imagery is, how it works, and the many ways it can support healing and recovery.

What Guided Imagery is:

A gentle, intentional practice that uses your imagination — through sights, sounds, sensations, and emotions — to create calming and healing experiences in your mind.

Similar to daydreaming, but with a purpose: helping your body relax, repair, and restore.

How it works:

Activates the mind-body connection: thoughts and images influence your nervous system, hormones, and immune system.

Triggers the relaxation response: slowing heart rate, lowering blood pressure, releasing muscle tension, and balancing stress hormones.

Engages the brain as if the imagined experience were real: visual, auditory, and motor areas light up during imagery.

Supports healing processes: may improve wound healing, reduce pain, and strengthen immune activity.

Provides a "healing blueprint": clear mental images of recovery give the body a positive script to follow.

Practical benefits and applications:

- Before surgery: reduces anxiety, promotes restful sleep, and helps patients mentally rehearse a smooth procedure.

- After surgery: supports healing, eases pain, and helps shorten recovery.

- Pain management: reduces distress and muscle tension, shifts focus away from discomfort, and gives patients a greater sense of control.

- Anxiety and stress relief: fosters calm and emotional balance in both medical and everyday settings.

- Recovery from illness or injury: maintains hope and positivity during the healing process.

- Living with chronic conditions: provides ongoing support for coping, rest, and resilience.

- Rehabilitation and wellness: pairs well with physical therapy, athletic training, and holistic practices like yoga and meditation.

Key takeaway: Guided imagery is a safe, versatile tool that can be used before, during, and after surgery, as well as in the event of illness or injury, and in daily life. Guided imagery doesn't replace medical care, but it is a powerful complement that helps the body and mind work together in healing.

Questions for Reflection

1. When you think about healing, what images naturally come to mind?

2. How do you currently use your imagination — and could you guide it more intentionally?

3. What does "healing" mean to you at this stage of your journey?

Part II – Evidence, Risks, and Rewards

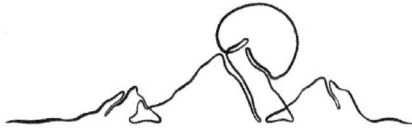

"The greatest weapon against stress is our ability to choose one thought over another."

-William James

Chapter 4 – What the Research Says

Guided imagery is a simple technique, but it has been studied for more than three decades in hospitals, clinics, and research centers. While results vary, the overall picture is encouraging: guided imagery can reduce anxiety, ease pain, and in some cases support faster recovery after surgery.

Surgery Preparation

Studies show that patients who practiced guided imagery before surgery often report less anxiety and feel more prepared.

In some trials, guided imagery reduced the need for sedatives before surgery.

Patients who imagined a smooth operation and recovery sometimes had shorter hospital stays and used less pain medication afterward.

Pain Management

Many studies find that guided imagery helps reduce the intensity of pain.

24

Patients often say they feel more in control of their pain when they use imagery.

Guided imagery is especially helpful when combined with other relaxation techniques, like slow breathing or progressive muscle relaxation.

Healing and Recovery

Some research suggests guided imagery may support the body's healing response by lowering stress hormones and improving immune function.

For example, patients who practiced imagery after surgery sometimes showed signs of faster wound healing and less fatigue.

The effects can differ depending on the type of surgery and how often imagery is practiced.

Emotional Well-Being

Guided imagery has been shown to reduce fear and worry before procedures.

Patients often describe feeling calmer, more confident, and better able to cope with recovery.

What We Don't Yet Know

Research is still mixed on outcomes like reducing complications, blood loss, or postoperative ileus (temporary slowing of the bowels).

Not every study finds large differences between guided imagery and usual care.

More high-quality research is needed, but current evidence strongly supports its role as a safe, low-cost tool for reducing stress and improving comfort.

Chapter 5 – Risks and Safety

One of the best things about guided imagery is its safety. Unlike medication or surgery, it carries very little risk. Still, it's important to know what to expect and how to use it wisely.

The Benefits Outweigh the Risks

- Non-invasive: Guided imagery requires no equipment and can be done almost anywhere.

- Safe for most people: Children, adults, and older adults can all practice it with ease.

- Low cost: Many recordings are free, and once you learn the skill, you can guide yourself.

Potential Challenges

- Emotional triggers: Sometimes imagery can stir up unexpected feelings, especially if a script includes scenes that don't feel safe or comforting.

- Difficulty visualizing: Not everyone "sees" images easily. Some may imagine through sounds, sensations, or feelings instead — and that's perfectly fine.

- Unrealistic expectations: Guided imagery is not a magic cure. It supports healing but does not replace medical treatment.

When to Use Extra Care

If you have a history of trauma, anxiety disorders, or severe depression, some imagery may feel unsettling. It may help to work with a trained therapist or use very gentle, neutral scripts.

If you feel uncomfortable at any point, you can always stop the exercise and return when you feel ready.

Bottom Line

Guided imagery is generally very safe. The main "risk" is disappointment if you expect it to do more than it can. Think of it as a supportive partner to your medical care — not a replacement for it.

Part II Summary

In this section, we explored both the research evidence and the safety profile of guided imagery.

What the research shows:

- Strong evidence supports guided imagery for reducing pre-surgery anxiety and easing post-surgery pain.

- Many patients also experience better emotional well-being and feel more in control.

- Some studies suggest improvements in recovery, wound healing, and reduced medication use, though results vary.

Risks and limitations:

- Guided imagery is safe and non-invasive, with no serious side effects reported.

- Some people may feel emotional discomfort if a script is unsettling or triggering, but this can be managed by choosing or creating imagery that feels safe and supportive.

- Guided imagery should never be seen as a replacement for medical care — only as a helpful addition.

Key takeaway: Guided imagery is a simple, safe, and effective tool that you can use before and after surgery, during recovery, or in daily life to reduce stress and support healing. The research is promising, and the risks are minimal.

Questions for Reflection

1. How do you usually respond to stress?

2. Can you recall a time when shifting your thoughts changed how you felt in your body?

3. What feels reassuring about knowing there's research supporting guided imagery?

Part III – Getting Started with Guided Imagery

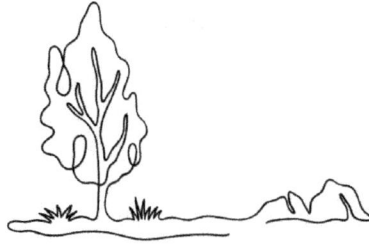

"When we give ourselves the chance to let go of all our tension, the body's natural capacity to heal itself can begin to work."

-Thich Nhat Hanh

Chapter 6 – Preparing for Practice

Before you begin guided imagery, a little preparation can make the experience smoother and more effective. Think of it as setting the foundation for relaxation.

Choosing the Right Time and Place

Create a do-not-disturb zone: Find a quiet space where you can be comfortable and relaxed, and tell family and housemates to leave you undisturbed for the duration of your practice. Silence smartphone notifications.

Many people practice before bed, first thing in the morning, or right before a medical appointment.

Over time, your body will start to recognize this time as "imagery time," making it easier to slip into relaxation.

Body Position and Comfort

Guided imagery can be done seated or lying down. If you choose to sit, keep both feet flat on the floor. If lying down, you may want to put a pillow under your knees to avoid straining your lower back.

Loosen tight clothing and adjust blankets or pillows for support.

Let your body feel safe and settled. Feel free to move and reposition yourself at any time if needed.

Setting an Intention

Before you start, pause for a moment and ask yourself: "What do I need most right now?" It may be calm, strength, healing, or courage. Allow that intention to guide your imagery.

Tools That Can Help

You can use headphones or speakers - try both and see which you prefer.

Using an eye mask or eye pillow will facilitate relaxation and may improve concentration.

Consider journaling or drawing afterward to deepen your practice.

Remember: even if conditions aren't perfect — maybe the hospital is noisy, or you only have a few minutes — guided imagery can still be effective.

Chapter 7 – How to Perform Guided Imagery

Now that you're prepared, we'll talk about guided imagery is done.

Always keep in mind that you can pause or stop a guided imagery session at any time if you feel any emotional or physical discomfort.

Step 1 – Begin with the Breath

Bringing awareness to the breath is how to begin any mind-body practice.

Begin by focusing your awareness on the feeling of breathing in your body. Bodily sensations that you may notice include your belly rising and falling, your ribcage expanding and contracting, and the coolness of the air as you inhale through your nostrils.

Take several slow, deep breaths.

Breathing calms the nervous system and signals your body that it's time to relax.

Step 2 – Close Your Eyes or Soften Your Gaze

This helps you turn your attention inward and focus on your inner world.

Step 3 - Scan and Relax Your Body

Briefly scan your body and release any tension that you may feel.

You can start with the feet and move upward, start with your head and move downward, or do one side of your body and then the other. Choose a method that feels and works best for you.

Step 4 – Engage the Senses

Guided imagery is about more than just visualizing images. Using all of your senses helps you create a more vivid and powerful scene.

Imagine:

- Environment: What time of day is it? What is the season? Are you inside or outside?

- Visuals: What do you see? Colors, shapes, furniture, landscapes?

- Sounds: Wind, waves, birds, soft music, or even silence.

- Touch: Coolness, warmth, textures, skin.

- Smell: Fresh air, flowers, or soothing aromas.

- Emotion: Peace, safety, or joy.

Step 5 - Follow a Script or Recording

You may:

- Use one of the scripts in this book.

- Listen to a recording from a trusted source.

- Guide yourself through your own chosen images.

Step 6 - Return Gently

When the imagery feels complete, slowly bring your attention back. Wiggle your fingers and toes, open your eyes, and take a final deep breath.

Self-Guided vs. Recorded Guidance

Recorded sessions are great for beginners — you just follow along.

Self-guided practice allows flexibility. Once you're comfortable, you can tailor imagery to your own needs.

There's no right or wrong way — choose whichever feels most supportive.

Part III Summary

In this section, you learned how to prepare and practice guided imagery.

Preparation matters: A quiet space, comfortable position, and a clear intention set the stage for success.

The practice is simple: Breathe, soften your gaze, relax your body, engage your senses, and follow a script or recording.

Flexibility is key: Even short, imperfect moments of practice can be powerful.

The choice is yours: use recordings when you want guidance, or lead yourself once you feel confident.

Key takeaway: Guided imagery is easy to begin. With just a few minutes, a comfortable place, and an open mind, you can start using it as a tool for relaxation and healing.

Questions for Reflection

1. What gets in the way of giving yourself time to rest and reset?

2. Where in your daily routine could you carve out five minutes for guided imagery?

3. What would it feel like to give yourself permission to pause?

Part IV – Enhancing Guided Imagery

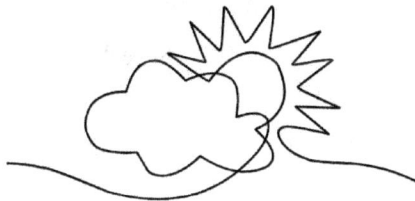

"Imagination is everything. It is the preview of life's coming attractions."

-Albert Einstein

Chapter 8 – Complementary Practices

Guided imagery is powerful on its own, but it can be even more effective when paired with other mind-body practices. Think of these as "companions" that make the imagery experience richer and more immersive.

Progressive Muscle Relaxation

Progressive muscle relaxation is a technique where you relax the body one part at a time. This technique is great for easing physical tension, calming anxiety, and improving sleep.

There are two ways to do progressive relaxation: Tensing and releasing each muscle group, or bringing awareness to the muscle group and releasing any felt tension.

Releasing physical tension helps your mind focus more easily on imagery. Imagining warmth or light spreading through your body as your muscles relax is also a great way to pair progressive relaxation and imagery.

Music and Sound

Soothing background music or natural sounds (waves, birdsong, rain) can help deepen relaxation.

Music can help block distracting noise in hospitals or waiting rooms.

Choose sounds that feel comforting and not overstimulating.

Aromatherapy

The chemical compounds in essential oils (the ingredients used in aromatherapy) stimulate neurons in the limbic system - the part of your brain responsible for regulating emotion, behavior, and memory. This is how aromatherapy can evoke strong emotions and trigger long-forgotten memories. These effects are rapid and can be both positive and negative.

Essential oils known to support relaxation and reduce anxiety include

- Lavender (*Lavandula angustifolia*)
- Sweet Orange (*Citrus sinensis*)
- Bergamot (*Citrus bergamia*)
- Roman Chamomile (*Chamaemelum nobile*)
- Frankincense (*Boswellia carterii*)
- Clary Sage (*Salvia sclarea*)
- Ylang Ylang (*Cananga odorata*)

- Vetiver (*Vetiveria zizanoides*)

Inhaling one of these oils, a blend, or any other scent that's relaxing or meaningful for you may improve and enhance your imagery session.

Use of a personal device (a drop on a cotton ball, a personal diffuser, a roller ball, or an aroma patch) is the quickest and easiest way to incorporate aromatherapy during an imagery session.

If you choose to use a room spray or room diffuser, be considerate of anyone else who might be exposed to the vapors - especially pets and sensitive individuals, including children and the elderly.

Always check for sensitivities or hospital restrictions before using any aromatherapy device.

Create a Personal Aroma Patch to Use During Guided Imagery

Here's a quick and easy way to create a personal aroma patch you can use during your guided imagery practice.

- Roll an adhesive bandage onto itself (inside-out), exposing the inner pad.

- Place 1-2 drops of essential oil on the pad.

- Secure the sticky part of the bandage to your clothing, close enough to your face so that you can inhale the vapors.

- Your patch should last for up to 12 hours.

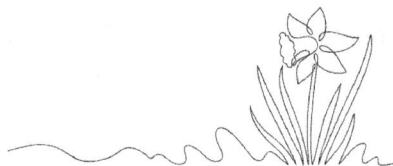

Chapter 9 – Using Affirmations

Affirmations are positive statements that you repeat to yourself. They are stated in the first person and in the present tense, such as "I am healthy and strong."

Affirmations are a great way to support your health and well-being and overcome undesirable habits and negative thinking. Affirmations provide strength and reassurance.

Using affirmations will enhance guided imagery, especially if you choose affirmations that reflect the positive imagery in your guided practice. Repetition builds new mental pathways, making healing imagery more powerful.

Affirmations can be used in many ways, such as writing them down, memorizing them for repeated use, or listening to pre-recorded audio. Listening to recorded affirmations can be done while doing other activities such as walking, housework, or even driving, because focus and stillness are not required to reap the benefits of this practice.

Affirmations For Healing and Recovery:

- I inhale peace and exhale fear and worry.

- My body heals naturally and fully.

- I take good care of my body.

- I release all fear and worry.

- I am aware of my breathing.

- I am healthy and whole.

- I heal from the inside out.

- I trust my body's wisdom and ability to heal.

- I free my mind from negative thoughts.

Chapter 10 – Strengthening Your Imagery and Visualization Skills

Some people see images clearly in their mind, while others imagine through sound, sensation, or emotion. Guided imagery works in all of these ways.

You can enhance and improve your visualization and imagery skills by incorporating these exercises and practices.

Of course, consistency and repetition are the best ways to strengthen your guided imagery practice!

Exercises to Enhance Visualization

Color Practice: Close your eyes and picture a single color, as vividly as you can.

Memory Recall: Think of a favorite place — what do you see, hear, and feel there?

Five Senses Exercise: Imagine holding a fruit. Picture its color, smell its aroma, feel its texture, imagine the taste and sound of biting into it.

Improving Your Ability to Visualize

Like any other skill, visualization can be improved with effort and practice. If you find it challenging to develop scenes and places in your imagination, trying one or two (or all!) of the following suggestions may help you improve your ability and confidence with visualization.

Find pictures of scenes or places that provoke a sense of peace, calm, or relaxation. Two good sources are magazines and calendars. Cut these images out and create a collection or collage to refer to when imagining yourself relaxing or resting peacefully.

Find a place in nature, such as a park or garden, where you can sit and relax. Look around at your surroundings and focus on all the sounds, sensations, and scents you see, hear, feel, and smell - taking them in and experiencing them fully and deeply. You may want to write a journal about your experience to recall it more vividly later.

Write a few paragraphs about a place, real or imagined, where you feel calm, relaxed, comfortable, and at peace. Include as many details as you can think of or remember.

Refer to this writing and continue to develop it with additional details each time you revisit it.

Chapter 11 – Developing an Inner Advisor

Most people have had at least one experience of having had a dream, insight, hunch, vision, or answer to a prayer that enlightened and guided them to deal with a challenging situation or decision. This form of intuition, or "knowing without knowing," often comes from deep within our subconscious.

The subconscious mind holds a vast amount of information - absorbing and remembering everything happening within and around us. Through imagery and visualization, you can develop your ability to call upon your subconscious and use this information to better understand yourself, your needs, and how you can meet them.

One way of calling on your subconscious is to develop an "inner advisor." An inner advisor is a wise, supportive figure you can meet during guided imagery. It may appear as a person, an animal, a light, or simply a sense of knowing.

Why Develop an Inner Advisor?

- Offers guidance when you feel uncertain.

- Provides comfort and reassurance during healing.

- Helps strengthen your sense of trust in yourself.

How to Connect with Your Inner Advisor

- Begin with relaxation and imagery.

- Imagine entering a safe, peaceful place.

- Invite your inner advisor to appear in whatever form feels right.

- Ask a simple question like, "What do I need most right now?"

- Listen or notice any images, words, or feelings that arise.

Over time, this practice can improve interoception — your awareness of what is happening in your body — and help you tune into your own inner wisdom.

Part IV Summary

In this section, you explored ways to deepen and personalize guided imagery:

Complementary practices like relaxation, music, and aromatherapy make imagery richer and easier.

Affirmations strengthen positive expectations and help replace fear with confidence.

Visualization skills improve with practice, and can be sharpened with simple exercises.

Inner advisors connect you with your own inner wisdom, offering comfort, clarity, and support.

Key takeaway: Guided imagery is flexible and adaptable. You can enrich it with affirmations, music, scents, and inner guidance — making the practice uniquely your own.

Questions for Reflection

1. Which senses (sight, sound, touch, smell, taste) feel strongest for you when you imagine?

2. What kinds of music, scents, or relaxation practices help you feel calm?

3. How might adding these supports make guided imagery easier or more enjoyable?

Part V – Guided Imagery Scripts

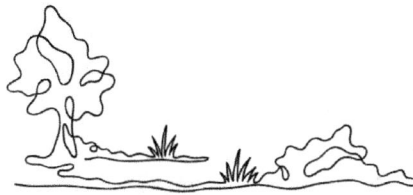

"Visualization is daydreaming with a purpose."

-Bo Bennett

How to Use These Scripts

The following guided imagery scripts are designed to help you relax, prepare for surgery, recover with confidence, and stay calm during medical procedures. You can use them on your own, with a trusted friend or caregiver, or as a recorded practice. Here are some tips to get the most out of them:

Go at Your Own Pace

Read the script slowly, then take yourself through your own guided imagery practice.

Don't try to recall and repeat everything you just read; use the script as a guide and inspiration.

Pause when you want more time with an image or sensation.

There's no "right" way to do this — allow the imagery to unfold naturally.

Adapt the Words

Feel free to edit these scripts as you see fit. If you prefer a different image, phrase, or affirmation, feel free to substitute.

I am grateful to have a body with two legs, two arms, two feet, two hands, and all five senses. The scripts included in this book are not meant to exclude anyone whose body may be different from mine, so please make any adjustments needed to adapt the script to suit your body and your needs.

The most important thing is that the imagery feels comforting and meaningful to you.

Make Your Own Recording

You can record yourself reading the script slowly, or ask a friend to do so.

When recording or reading out loud, speak slowly and with a soft, normal voice, but not a whisper.

Three dots (...) indicate where you may want to take a breath or pause for three to five seconds. This will help you create a recording that sounds soothing and relaxing, without distracting you from the practice.

Pairing recordings with gentle background music or nature sounds can enhance the experience.

These scripts are tools to support you — before surgery, during recovery, or whenever you want to relax. Use them flexibly, adapt them to your needs, and let them become part of your healing routine.

A reminder: These guided imagery practices are intended for relaxation and support only. They are not a substitute for medical care or treatment. If you have any health concerns, please consult your doctor before beginning.

Chapter 12 – Relaxation and Healing

This script is designed for times when you want to relax deeply and support your body's natural healing process. You can use it before or after surgery, while recovering from illness or injury, or simply at the end of a stressful day. It is especially helpful when you are feeling tense, restless, or overwhelmed, as it helps calm both the mind and the body. Even if you only have a few minutes, this practice can restore balance and create a sense of comfort and renewal.

See the resources section for the link to a recording of this script, available for free on Soundcloud.

Script for Relaxation and Healing

Find a comfortable position - seated or lying down, ankles and legs uncrossed. Palms up, arms resting lightly at your sides or in your lap.

Allow your eyes to close softly. Take in a slow, gentle breath, inhaling through the nose, then slowly exhale through your nose or mouth...

Continue to breathe softly and slowly, allowing your breath to flow naturally and with ease...

Feel your body begin to soften - your soft belly rising and falling with each inhale and exhale. With each breath, allow your body to soften a little more...

Feel your feet relax... Feel your hands relax. Allow your hands and feet to become warm and heavy... Feel your shoulders ease and your jaw relax. Relax your forehead. Continue to breathe in and out of your belly button...

Now imagine yourself in a place of peace and comfort — maybe a beach at sunrise, a quiet and peaceful room, a beautiful forest clearing, or a garden filled with light...

Notice the details of this place you've chosen: What is the time of day? What is the season? Is it light or dark or somewhere in between?...

What objects do you see around you, near or far? Notice shapes, colors, and textures of anything you can see...

Notice the feeling of your clothing or anything touching your skin...the temperature of the air - any warmth or coolness that you may feel on your skin...

Notice any sounds you hear here - maybe it's silence, that's okay...

Notice any smells you may smell in this place. Imagine and name any smells you might find here...

Allow yourself to feel safe and supported in this space...

As you rest here, picture a warm, healing light surrounding you...

With each breath in, this light fills your body, moving gently around and through every cell of your body.... With each breath out, you release tension, worry, fear, or discomfort...

Focus on the color and intensity of this healing light. Allow the light to pulsate and flow in rhythm with your breath...

Notice if the light emits any sound, or scent...

Now let the light settle wherever your body most needs healing. Allow the light to soothe any areas of discomfort, release tension, calm your heart, relax your lungs, and strengthen your immune system...

Trust that your body knows how and where to use this healing energy…

Repeat quietly to yourself:

"I am calm and at peace."

"I feel supported."

"My body is healing."

Stay with this peaceful scene for as long as you wish...

When you're ready to emerge from this practice, gently bring your awareness back to your surroundings, taking one or two deep breaths. Wiggle your fingers and toes. Gently open your eyes.

Continue carrying this sense of healing with you.

Chapter 13 – The Ideal Surgery and Recovery Experience

This script is meant for the days or weeks leading up to surgery. It helps you prepare mentally and emotionally by imagining a smooth, safe procedure and a steady, confident recovery. Patients often find that practicing this imagery reduces anxiety, improves sleep before surgery, and helps them feel more trust in their care team. Use this script whenever you notice worry about your upcoming procedure, or as part of your daily routine as the surgery date approaches.

Script for Visualizing the Ideal Surgery and Recovery Experience

Find a quiet, comfortable place where you can sit or lie down. Allow your eyes to softly close. Take in a slow, gentle breath, inhaling through the nose, then slowly exhale through your nose or mouth...

Continue to breathe softly and slowly, allowing your breath to flow naturally and with ease...

Feel your body begin to soften - your soft belly rising and falling with each inhale and exhale. With each breath, allow your body to soften a little more...

Feel your feet relax... Feel your hands relax. Allow your hands and feet to become warm and heavy... Feel your shoulders ease and your jaw relax. Relax your forehead. Continue to breathe in and out of your belly button...

Now imagine yourself waking up the morning of your surgery. Imagine feeling rested and relaxed as you get up and get ready to have your surgery...

Picture yourself arriving at the hospital or clinic, feeling calm and supported. See the staff welcoming you, greeting you with kindness, guiding you gently through each step...

Visualize yourself in the pre-op area. Changing into your hospital gown, lying on the stretcher, feeling warm and comfortable under the covers...

See yourself remaining calm and relaxed as the staff prepares you for your procedure...

Visualize the operating room as a place of safety. The team works with skill and focus, every detail unfolding smoothly. Imagine yourself resting peacefully, your body responding exactly as it should...

Visualize your body remaining relaxed and steady during the procedure. Your body begins the healing process immediately...

Now picture your recovery. Imagine waking up, feeling comfortable, breathing easily, and sensing that healing has already begun...See your body knitting itself back together — stronger, healthier, whole...

Affirm silently:

"I trust my body."

"I trust my care team."

"I recover with ease and confidence."

Stay with this sense of trust and healing for a few breaths...

When you're ready to emerge from this practice, gently bring your awareness back to your surroundings, taking one or two deep breaths. Wiggle your fingers and toes. Gently open your eyes.

Continue carrying this sense of trust and healing with you.

Chapter 14 – Reducing Fear and Anxiety During a Brief Medical Procedure

This script is designed to help you stay calm and steady during quick but sometimes stressful medical moments, such as an IV start, epidural placement, blood draw, or injection. It's handy for when you feel nervous in a clinic or hospital setting and need fast relief. By focusing on your breath and a safe mental image, you can shift your attention away from fear and anchor yourself in calm, even if the procedure lasts only a few minutes.

Script for Reducing Fear and Anxiety During a Brief Medical Procedure

Take a slow breath in through your nose … and exhale gently through your mouth. Feel your shoulders drop as you let go of tension.

Bring to mind a safe, comforting place — perhaps sitting by a fire, resting under a tree, or wrapped in a warm blanket. Let yourself feel secure there.

As you focus on this image, repeat silently with each breath:

Inhale: "I am calm."

Exhale: "I am safe."

If you notice fear rising, imagine releasing it with your breath, like a dark cloud drifting away. With each inhale, picture strength and comfort filling you.

As the procedure begins, stay anchored in your breath and your safe image. Remind yourself: "This moment will pass quickly. I am steady. I am strong."

When it is finished, take one more slow breath and gently return to your surroundings, carrying calm with you.

Part V Summary

In this section, you practiced three guided imagery scripts designed for different situations:

Relaxation and Healing — to reduce stress, encourage rest, and support the body's natural healing processes.

Ideal Surgery and Recovery — to prepare for surgery with calm confidence and visualize smooth recovery.

Reducing Fear During Brief Procedures — to stay grounded and calm during short but stressful medical events.

Key takeaway: Guided imagery can be tailored to your needs. Whether you have hours to prepare or only a few minutes in a hospital room, you can use your imagination and breath to create calm, confidence, and healing from within.

Questions for Reflection

1. How do you usually "see" things in your mind — clearly, vaguely, or more through feelings?

2. What script feels most relevant to your situation right now: relaxation, surgery prep, or easing fear?

3. How could you make the words and images in a script feel more personal to you?

Part VI - Practical Tools for Your Journey

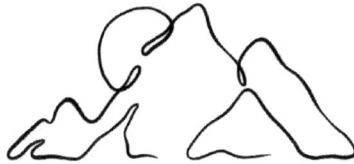

"The future depends on what you do today."

-Mahatma Gandhi

In the earlier parts of this book, you explored the background, science, and benefits of guided imagery for healing. Now, it's time to move from understanding to action. Consider this section your toolkit — a collection of practical advice, exercises, and worksheets designed to help you bring guided imagery into your daily life.

Here, you'll find simple strategies for practicing in different settings, guidance for overcoming common challenges, and step-by-step prompts for creating your own personalized imagery. These tools are meant to be flexible — you can use them as stand-alone practices or combine them with the scripts and techniques already introduced.

Think of Part VI as your hands-on guidebook: a place to return to whenever you want inspiration, structure, or a reminder that even small moments of guided imagery today can shape your healing tomorrow.

Chapter 15 - Doing Guided Imagery in Public Places

Guided imagery can be done almost anywhere, even in a busy environment like a waiting room, hospital hallway, or during a commute. Here are some tips to make the practice easier and more comfortable in public spaces:

Find a Semi-Quiet Spot

Look for a corner, an empty bench, or even a seat near a window.

Noise is okay — you don't need silence for guided imagery to work.

Use Headphones

Play a recorded script or soothing background sounds through headphones or earbuds.

Headphones create a personal bubble and signal to others that you don't want to be disturbed.

Choose a Comfortable Posture

Sit with your feet on the ground and hands resting in your lap.

Keep your body language relaxed but natural so you don't feel self-conscious.

Soften Your Focus

You don't have to close your eyes if that feels awkward. Instead, let your gaze rest on the floor or a neutral spot.

Some people find it easier to look out a window or at a calming image on their phone.

Keep It Short and Simple

A 2–5 minute practice is enough in public settings.

Focus on a single image, like walking on a beach, sitting under a tree, or breathing in healing light.

Use the Breath as an Anchor

If distractions pull you away, gently return to your breath.

Inhale calm, exhale tension — repeat this as your background rhythm.

Adapt Your Script

Instead of long, detailed imagery, choose one or two comforting images.

Example: "With each breath, I imagine a soft wave of calm moving through me."

End Smoothly

Take a final deep breath and gently reorient to your surroundings.

Open your eyes fully, stretch, or look around before resuming your activity.

A Quick Script for Doing Guided Imagery in a Public Place

Take a slow breath in through your nose ... and a gentle breath out through your mouth.

Let your shoulders soften. Feel your body supported where you sit.

Now imagine a wave of calm moving gently through you with each breath.

As you breathe in, picture light and peace filling your body.

As you breathe out, imagine releasing any tension or worry.

Bring to mind a simple, comforting image — maybe a favorite tree, a warm beam of sunlight, or a calm shoreline. Hold that picture softly in your mind.

Repeat silently to yourself: "I am calm. I am safe. My body is healing."

Take one more steady breath in ... and a slow breath out. When you're ready, return to your surroundings, carrying this calm with you.

Chapter 16 - The Role of Breathing in Mind-Body Practices

Breathing is the bridge between the body and the mind. It happens automatically, but when we bring awareness to our breath, it becomes a powerful tool for relaxation, focus, and healing.

Why Breath Matters

Your breath is a direct link to your nervous system. Slow, steady breathing activates the parasympathetic nervous system (the "rest and digest" response), calming the body and reducing stress.

Foundation for relaxation:

Almost every mind-body practice — guided imagery, meditation, yoga, progressive relaxation — begins with focusing on the breath.

Anchor for attention:

Your breath is always with you. Focusing on it helps you quiet your mind and brings your awareness to the present moment.

Support for healing:

Deep, relaxed breathing improves oxygen flow, lowers blood pressure, eases muscle tension, and creates a state of balance that supports the body's natural healing processes.

Simple Breathing Techniques to Try

Slow Counting Breath

Inhale gently to the count of four.

Exhale slowly to the count of six.

Repeat for a few cycles, noticing how your body softens.

Belly Breathing (Diaphragmatic Breathing)

Place both hands over your belly.

Take a slow, deep breath in, feeling your belly rise.

As you breathe out, feel your belly fall.

Repeat for a few breaths.

This quickly shifts your body into relaxation mode.

Sigh of Relief

Take a slow breath in.

Exhale with an audible sigh.

Feel tension melting away as you let go.

Quick Reminders

Always inhale through the nose - this automatically activates the diaphragm and leads to a deeper, fuller breath.

Even one or two deep breaths can change how you feel.

You don't need to force the breath — gentle and natural is best.

Pairing breathing with guided imagery strengthens both practices.

Your breath is your most accessible healing tool. By learning to slow it down and pay attention to it, you create the perfect foundation for guided imagery and other mind-body practices.

Chapter 17 - Common Challenges in Guided Imagery

Most people find guided imagery relaxing and helpful, but it's normal to run into a few challenges, especially when you're first starting. Here are some common experiences and tips for handling them:

Feeling Overwhelmed

Sometimes imagery can stir up uncomfortable emotions. You may feel sadness, worry, or even frustration.

Tip: Remind yourself you are in control — you can always pause, open your eyes, or switch to a more neutral image (like focusing only on your breath).

If overwhelming feelings happen often, consider using very simple imagery (like imagining light or a safe place) or working with a trained professional.

Falling Asleep

Because guided imagery is deeply relaxing, it's common to drift off.

Tip: If you want to stay awake, try sitting upright instead of lying down, or practice earlier in the day when you have more energy.

If you do fall asleep, don't worry — your body still benefits from the relaxation.

Physical Discomfort

You may notice restlessness, muscle tension, or difficulty finding a comfortable position.

Tip: Adjust your posture, use pillows or blankets for support, and don't hesitate to move during the practice. Guided imagery doesn't require stillness.

Even a few minutes of comfort will provide benefits.

These experiences are normal and not a sign of "doing it wrong." Guided imagery is flexible — you can adjust it so it feels safe, comfortable, and supportive for you.

Chapter 18 - Creating Your Ideal Surgery Visualization

Guided imagery is most powerful when it feels personal. While recordings and scripts can guide you, there is tremendous value in creating your own visualization. This process helps you explore what matters most to you, strengthens your sense of control, and creates a mental "blueprint" for the experience you want.

Why Create Your Own Visualization?

- Tailored to your procedure: Every surgery and every patient is different. You can shape your imagery around your exact situation — whether it's orthopedic, abdominal, gynecological, or another type of surgery.

- Strengthens intention: Writing your own words makes the visualization more vivid and believable to your mind and body.

- Empowers you: Actively imagining a positive outcome gives you a sense of participation in your healing process.

- Flexibility: You benefit from the process whether you listen to it later or not. The act of creating it is healing in itself.

Steps to Create Your Visualization

Before Surgery

Picture yourself arriving at the hospital feeling calm and supported.

Imagine your care team greeting you with kindness and professionalism.

See yourself being prepared for surgery smoothly and efficiently.

Affirm: "I am ready. I am safe. I trust my care team and my body."

During Surgery

Imagine your body cooperating with the surgical team, everything working in harmony.

You might include healing suggestions like:

"My body directs blood flow exactly where it needs to be, reducing unnecessary blood loss."

"My heart and lungs remain strong, steady, and calm."

Visualize your body as steady, efficient, and safe throughout the procedure.

Awakening from Surgery

See yourself waking calmly and comfortably, breathing smoothly and clearly.

Picture your digestive system coming back online — you may imagine the gentle gurgle of your stomach and bowels as a sign of recovery.

Affirm: "I awaken refreshed, comfortable, and ready to heal."

Recovery and Beyond

Imagine your incision healing neatly, with skin and tissue knitting together smoothly.

Visualize yourself regaining strength day by day, walking confidently, and returning to the activities you love.

Affirm: "Each day I grow stronger. Healing continues with every breath."

How to Capture Your Visualization

Write it down: Use a journal or notebook. Write in the present tense, as if it's already happening.

Use the worksheets provided in the next section: *Create Your Ideal Surgical Visualization* and *Quick Worksheet: Create Your Ideal Surgical Visualization*. All worksheets are available as PDFs for you to download, print, and use; a QR code to access links is provided in the Resources section.

Keep it positive: Focus on what you want to experience, not what you fear.

Use your senses: Include sights, sounds, feelings, and even smells or tastes to make it vivid.

Be specific: Tailor your imagery to your own surgery, health status, and personal healing goals.

Sharing Your Visualization

With your care team: Sharing your visualization with a nurse, anesthetist, or surgeon can help them understand your mindset and support you.

With loved ones: Reading it to family or friends can bring encouragement and help them visualize your healing, too.

With yourself: Reading it back, especially before bed, can reinforce calm and confidence.

By creating your own surgical visualization, you give your body a healing script to follow. Writing it down and practicing it is powerful on its own, whether or not you record it or listen back later. This is your story — your body, your surgery, your healing — and your visualization makes it uniquely yours.

Worksheets

A QR code to access links for PDFs of these worksheets can be found in the Resources section.

The worksheets in this section are designed to help you take guided imagery from an idea into a personal practice. Writing down your thoughts, intentions, and imagery makes the process more vivid and real — it helps your mind and body remember what you want to create for yourself.

Some worksheets will guide you step by step in creating your own surgical visualization. Others provide examples, quick prompts, or reflection questions you can return to as your healing journey continues. You do not have to complete them all at once. Instead, choose the worksheets that feel most relevant to your needs right now.

Think of these pages as a toolbox: use them to prepare before surgery, to reflect during recovery, or simply to support your well-being day to day. Whether you use them once or return to them again and again, these exercises will help you deepen your practice and strengthen your role as an active participant in your healing.

Worksheet: Create Your Ideal Surgical Visualization

Use this worksheet to create a personalized imagery script for your surgery. Write in the present tense, as if the experience is happening now. Keep it positive, simple, and tailored to your situation. Don't worry about making it "perfect." The act of imagining and writing is powerful on its own. Your visualization is your story — unique to you, your body, and your healing.

Step 1: Set Your Intention

What do you want most from this experience? (e.g., calm, confidence, healing, trust)

My intention for this visualization is:

Step 2: Before Surgery

Describe how you arrive and feel as you prepare for surgery.

Who greets you?

How does your body feel?

What words help you feel safe?

My imagery before surgery:

Step 3: During Surgery

Picture your body working smoothly with your care team.

How do you want your heart, lungs, and body systems to respond?

Imagine your body directing blood flow efficiently to reduce blood loss.

Visualize everything unfolding calmly and safely.

My imagery during surgery:

Step 4: Awakening After Surgery

Imagine how you wake up after the procedure.

How do you want to feel as you open your eyes?

What signs of recovery do you picture (steady breath, comfort, stomach gurgling, bowels waking up)?

What affirmations support you?

My imagery awakening after surgery:

Step 5: Recovery and Beyond

Visualize your healing journey after surgery.

How do your incision and tissues heal?

How do you regain strength, movement, and energy?

What do you picture yourself doing once you're well again?

My imagery for recovery:

Step 6: My Affirmations

Write 2–3 short, positive statements you'll repeat to yourself. (e.g., "I am safe." "My body heals with every breath.")

Step 7: Share and Practice

Write it down: Keep your script in a notebook or journal.

Share it: Read it to a loved one or member of your care team.

Practice it: Read it to yourself, especially before bed or in quiet moments.

Example Completed Worksheet: My Ideal Surgical Visualization

My intention for this visualization is:

"To stay calm, trust my care team, and heal smoothly and quickly."

My imagery before surgery:

"I arrive at the hospital feeling peaceful and supported. The staff greet me warmly and everything flows easily. As I wait, I take slow breaths and feel safe, knowing my body is strong and ready. I repeat to myself: 'I am calm, I am safe, I am ready.'"

My imagery during surgery:

"My body works in harmony with my doctors and nurses. My blood flows efficiently and only where it's needed, reducing blood loss. My heart and lungs remain steady and calm. My body is strong and resilient, doing exactly what it needs to for a smooth surgery."

My imagery awakening after surgery:

"I wake up gently, breathing easily and feeling comfortable. I notice a calm gurgle in my stomach as my digestive system begins to wake up. I feel light, refreshed, and relieved that the surgery is complete. I tell myself: 'I awaken with peace, comfort, and healing energy.'"

My imagery for recovery:

"My incision heals quickly, with the skin and tissue coming together neatly. Each day I feel stronger and more comfortable. I picture myself walking with ease, laughing with my family, and returning to the activities I love. Healing continues every day."

My Affirmations

I am safe and supported.

My body knows how to heal.

Each day I become stronger and more comfortable.

Share and Practice

I wrote my script in my journal.

I shared it with my partner, who reads it to me before bed.

I review it each night and each morning, reminding myself of my strength and calm.

Note to Reader: This is just an example — your words, your surgery, and your healing story will be unique.

Quick Worksheet: Create Your Ideal Surgical Visualization

This quick worksheet gives you the essential prompts to create your own surgical visualization. Write in the present tense, keep it positive, and focus on your healing and recovery.

Intention: What do I want most? (calm, healing, trust)

Before Surgery: How do I arrive? Who greets me? How do I feel safe?

During Surgery: My body works with the team. I direct blood flow. I stay steady.

Awakening: How do I wake up? Breathing, comfort, stomach gurgle, peace.

Recovery: My incision heals, I regain strength, I return to my life.

Affirmations: Write 2–3 positive statements (e.g., 'I am safe').

Practice: How will I share or repeat my visualization daily?

My Healing Plan Worksheet

Use this worksheet to reflect on your journey with guided imagery and create a personal healing plan. Take time to write your answers thoughtfully.

Looking Back: What are the three most important things I've learned from this book about guided imagery and healing?

Personal Tools: Which scripts, tips, or practices felt most useful to me — and why?

My Visualization: If I were to create one powerful healing image or scene that I can return to again and again, what would it look and feel like?

Daily Integration: When and where can I realistically practice guided imagery in my daily routine?

Support System: Who can I share my visualization or practice with — to help me feel encouraged and supported?

My Commitment: What is one small, specific step I can take today to begin (or continue) using guided imagery as part of my healing journey?

Closing Note on Worksheets

You've now explored a variety of worksheets designed to help you bring guided imagery into your daily life. Each exercise — whether it was a reflection prompt, a personalized surgical visualization, or your healing plan — is meant to give you a sense of ownership in your healing journey.

Remember, you don't have to do everything at once. Some days you may feel drawn to write in detail; other days, a few affirmations or a quick visualization may be all you need. The goal is not perfection — it's practice.

Return to these worksheets whenever you need focus, encouragement, or a reminder that you are an active participant in your healing. Even small moments of reflection can bring peace, strength, and direction.

Part VI Summary

In this section, you've explored a set of practical tools designed to make guided imagery a natural part of your daily life. From practicing quietly in public spaces, to using breath as an anchor, to working through common challenges, these strategies help you adapt guided imagery to real-world situations. You've also learned how to create your own personalized surgical visualization, giving you a way to prepare your mind and body with intention and confidence.

The worksheets provided — both detailed and condensed — offer a framework you can return to again and again. They are not only a way to plan your imagery, but also a means of deepening your relationship with your own healing process.

Most importantly, Part VI reminds you that healing is not just something that happens to you — it's something you can actively participate in. Each practice you choose, no matter how small, strengthens your ability to meet surgery, recovery, or illness with clarity, resilience, and hope.

Now, before moving on, take a few moments with the reflection questions below to consider how you'll weave these tools into your own journey.

Questions for Reflection

1. Which tool in this section feels most practical or helpful for me right now?

2. What challenges have I faced in the past when trying to relax or visualize, and how might I use the tips here to handle them differently?

3. What is one small step I can take today to make guided imagery a steady part of my healing journey?

Conclusion - Your Healing Journey

You've reached the end of this book, but this is just the beginning of your healing journey with guided imagery. Along the way, you've learned what guided imagery is, how it works, the research that supports it, and the many ways you can use it to ease anxiety, support recovery, and strengthen your sense of well-being. You've also discovered scripts, affirmations, and complementary practices that can make your imagery practice richer and more personal.

At its heart, guided imagery is simple: it's about giving your mind gentle, positive pictures to hold, so your body can respond with calm and healing. It's about creating space for peace in the middle of uncertainty, and reminding yourself that you have tools within you to meet challenges with steadiness and strength.

A Few Final Reminders

There's no one "right" way. Guided imagery is flexible. Adapt the words, images, and affirmations so they feel natural to you.

Practice is powerful. The more you use guided imagery — even for just a few minutes each day — the more easily your body will learn to relax and respond.

It's a partner, not a replacement. Guided imagery is meant to support, not substitute for, medical care. Use it alongside your treatments, medications, and the wisdom of your healthcare team.

Trust yourself. Your body knows how to heal. Your mind can help guide the way.

Carrying Guided Imagery Forward

Whether you're preparing for surgery, recovering from illness, or simply seeking more calm in daily life, guided imagery is a practice you can carry with you anywhere. It requires no special equipment, no long hours, and no perfect conditions — just your breath, your imagination, and your willingness to pause.

As you move forward, may you find comfort in your practice, courage in your healing, and peace in knowing that you have within you a powerful resource for well-being.

Final Reflection

Before you close this book, take a quiet moment to reflect on your journey. Guided imagery works best when it is personal, intentional, and practiced. Use these prompts to help you capture what matters most for your own healing.

Looking Back:

What are the three most important things I've learned from this book about guided imagery and healing?

Personal Tools:

Which scripts, tips, or practices felt most useful to me — and why?

My Visualization:

If I were to create one powerful healing image or scene that I can return to again and again, what would it look and feel like?

Daily Integration:

When and where can I realistically practice guided imagery in my daily routine? (For example: morning, before bed, waiting at the doctor's office.)

Support System:

Who can I share my visualization or practice with — to help me feel encouraged and supported?

My Commitment:

What is one small, specific step I can take today to begin (or continue) using guided imagery as part of my healing journey?

A Thought to Carry With You

Healing isn't a single event — it is a process. Guided imagery is one way of reminding yourself that you have the ability to bring calm, hope, and direction into that process. Whatever challenges you may face, know that the tools you carry within you are always available.

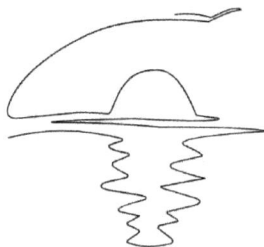

"The body achieves what the mind believes."

-Anonymous

Resources

Guided imagery is most effective when you have support and options that fit your needs.

Scan this OR code to access PDFs of worksheets and a curated collection of online resources, apps, books, and audiobooks for practice and further reading.

References

The following studies and reviews provide evidence for the use of guided imagery in surgery preparation, healing, and recovery.

Key Research Studies

Holden-Lund, C. (1988). Effects of relaxation with guided imagery on surgical stress and wound healing. Research in Nursing & Health.

Tusek, D. et al. (1997). Guided imagery: a significant advance in the care of patients undergoing elective colorectal surgery. Diseases of the Colon & Rectum.

Gonzales, E. et al. (2010). Effects of guided imagery on postoperative outcomes in same-day surgery. AORN Journal.

Charette, S. et al. (2015). Guided imagery for adolescent post-spinal fusion pain management: a pilot randomized controlled trial. Pain Management Nursing.

Zengin Aydın, L. & Doğan, A. (2023). Guided imagery and postoperative pain after lower-extremity surgery: randomized controlled trial.

Systematic Reviews

Álvarez-García, C. et al. (2020). Effects of preoperative guided imagery interventions: systematic review. International Journal of Nursing Studies Advances.

Anamagh, M. et al. (2024). Effect of guided imagery on perioperative anxiety in hospitalized adults: systematic review. Perioperative Care and Operating Room Management.

Rajjoub, R. et al. (2024). Meditation for perioperative pain and anxiety: systematic review. Annals of Medicine & Surgery.

Also by the Author

Mind-Body Practices for Surgery Support

A brief, practical online course that teaches breathing, relaxation, and imagery techniques to reduce anxiety and support healing before and after surgery. Includes video instruction and audio practices.

Available at: prepareforyoursurgery.thinkific.com

About the Author

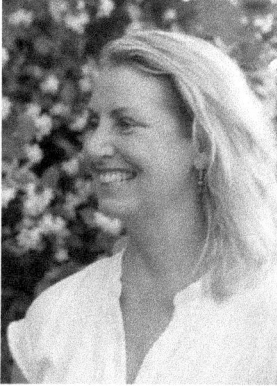

Becky Stevens is a nurse anesthetist and board-certified holistic nurse with over 30 years of experience in patient care. She specializes in teaching mind-body practices, such as guided imagery, to help patients reduce anxiety, ease pain, and support healing before and after surgery. Becky is passionate about empowering people to take an active role in their recovery by blending modern medicine with holistic, evidence-based practices.

Please visit her website **Prepareforyoursurgery.com** for more information about integrative health and wellness, her blog, and a curated collection of resources to help and guide you in your journey of health and healing.

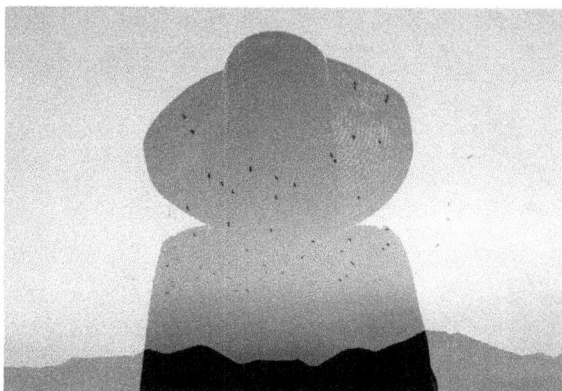

"When we work to heal ourselves, we contribute to healing of the whole."

-Jean Watson